x617
E£3f

Elgin, Kathleen
   The fall down, break a bone, skin your
knee, book. Written and illus. by
Kathleen Elgin. Walker 1974
   64p illus

   Explains some com... bruises, muscle sp... 3 1192 00043 6426
and nosebleeds.

1.Physiology 2.Accidents I.Title

AP   DATE DUE

OCT 1 6 1979

M
MA

X 133

Evanston Public Library
Evanston, Illinois

Each reader is responsible for all
books or other materials taken on his
card, and for any fines or fees
charged for overdues, damages, or
loss.

DEMCO

THE FALL
DOWN,
BREAK
A BONE,
SKIN YOUR KNEE BOOK

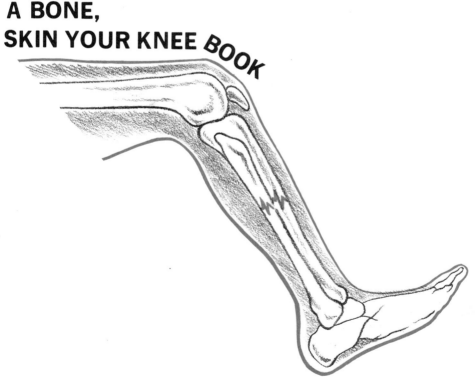

EVANSTON PUBLIC LIBRARY
CHILDREN'S DEPARTMENT
1703 ORRINGTON AVENUE
EVANSTON, ILLINOIS 60201

The Fall Down, Break a Bone, Skin Your Knee, BOOK

WRITTEN AND
ILLUSTRATED BY

KATHLEEN ELGIN

x617
El 3f

Bt176

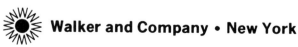 Walker and Company • New York

The author wishes to thank
John F. Osterrwitter, M.D., Ph.D.,
for giving a professional
appraisal of this book.

Copyright© 1974 by Kathleen Elgin

All rights reserved. No part of this book may be reproduced
or transmitted in any form or by any means, electronic or
mechanical, including photocopying, recording, or by any
information storage and retrieval system, without permission
in writing from the Publisher.

First published in the United States of America in 1974
by the Walker Publishing Company, Inc.

Published simultaneously in Canada by Fitzhenry
& Whiteside, Limited, Toronto.

Trade ISBN: 8027-6179-8
Reinf. ISBN: 8027-6180-1

Library of Congress Catalog Card Number: 73-92450

Printed in the United States of America.

10 9 8 7 6 5 4 3 2 1

Contents

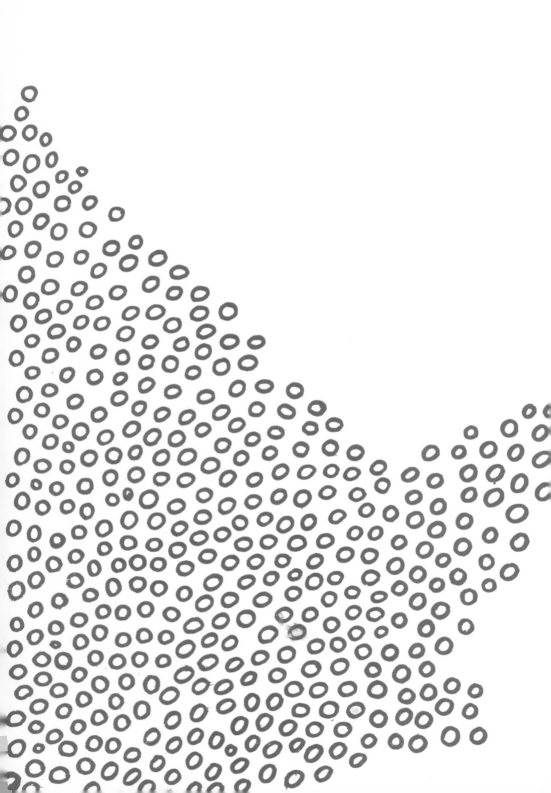

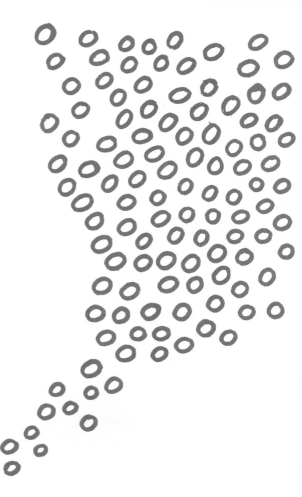

CELLS

You have trillions of *cells* in your body. There are cells in your bones, in your muscles and skin, and in your nerves. There are also cells in your blood and lungs, heart, stomach, and brain.

Your entire body is made up of many different cells.

A cell is a unit of living matter. It has two main parts: a *nucleus*, or cell headquarters, and the surrounding *cytoplasm*. A *cell membrane* encircles the jelly-like cytoplasm like a wall. It keeps the contents of the cell in place, and allows food and wastes to pass in and out.

Each tiny cell is an extremely busy chemical "factory." The nucleus controls the activity of the cytoplasm, where most of the cell's work is carried on.

The cytoplasm breaks down food which enters the cell through the cell membrane. It changes the food into energy for your body. It also manufactures more cytoplasm for growth.

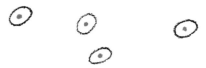

CYTOPLASM

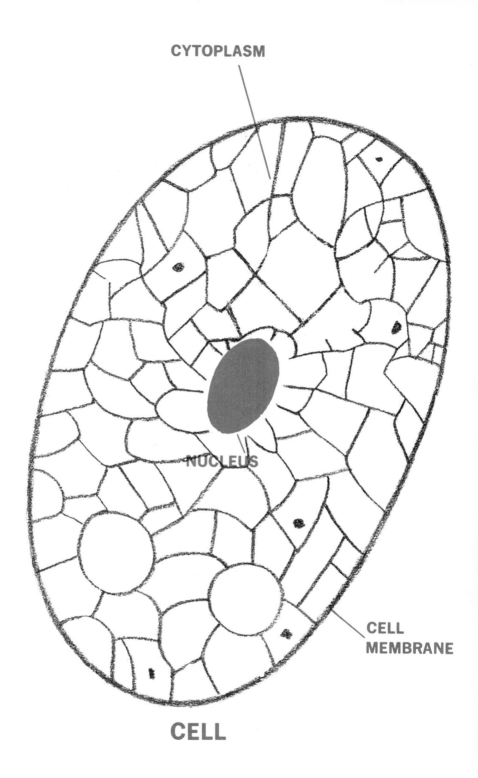

NUCLEUS

CELL
MEMBRANE

CELL

9

When many cells are joined together and do the same work, they are called *tissues*. There are different types of tissue—for example, bone, muscle, blood, skin, and connective tissue. Tissue cells are working, wearing out, and being constantly replaced every minute and every day of your life.

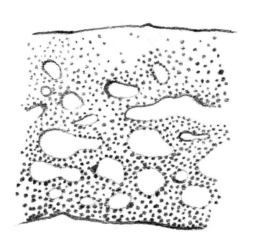

BONE TISSUE

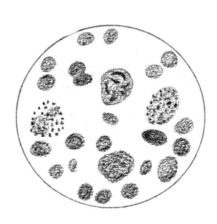

BLOOD TISSUE

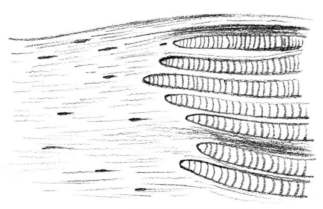

MUSCLE TISSUE

Sometimes, they have to rebuild faster than usual. If you fall off your bicycle and cut your knee, new skin tissue must be formed right away so that the cut can heal. If you break a bone playing a rough game of football, your bone cells have to work hard and fast to help your body repair the injury.

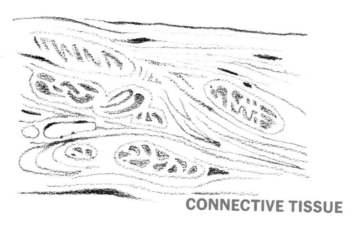

CONNECTIVE TISSUE

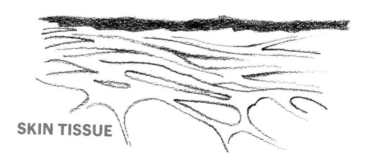

SKIN TISSUE

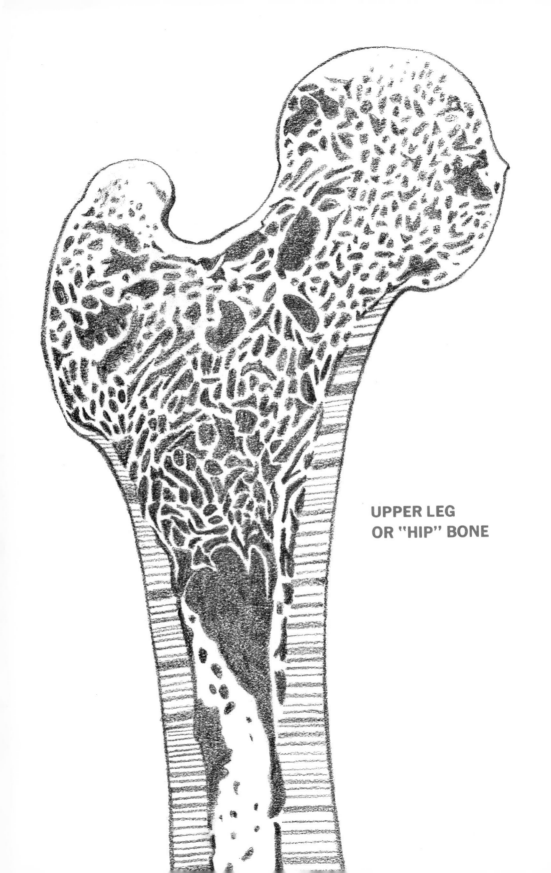

UPPER LEG
OR "HIP" BONE

BREAK A BONE

A bone is made up of bone tissue, which consists of living cells like any other tissue. Unlike other tissues, however, bone tissue is very hard. It is also very strong, and amazingly lightweight for all it has to support.

About one-half of bone tissue is made up of minerals such as *calcium* and *phosphorus*. About a quarter of the bone is *collagen*. Collagen comes from the Greek words "kolla" (glue) and "gene" (forming). The collagen cements together the minerals in the bone and gives it strength. Almost all the rest of the bone is water!

There are four different kinds of bone: long bones, short bones, flat bones, and irregular bones. Examples of these four kinds are:

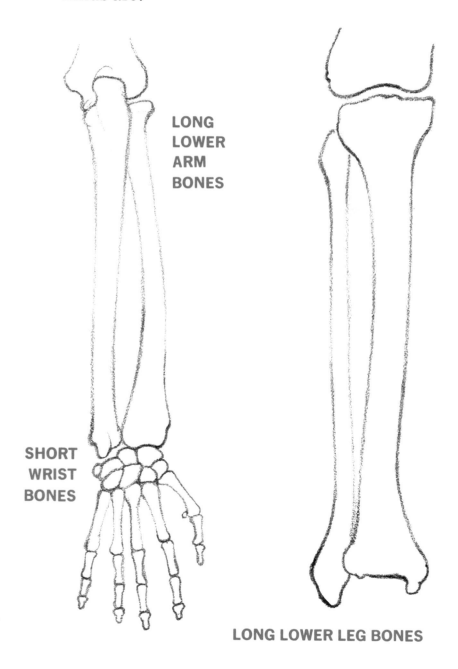

LONG LOWER ARM BONES

SHORT WRIST BONES

LONG LOWER LEG BONES

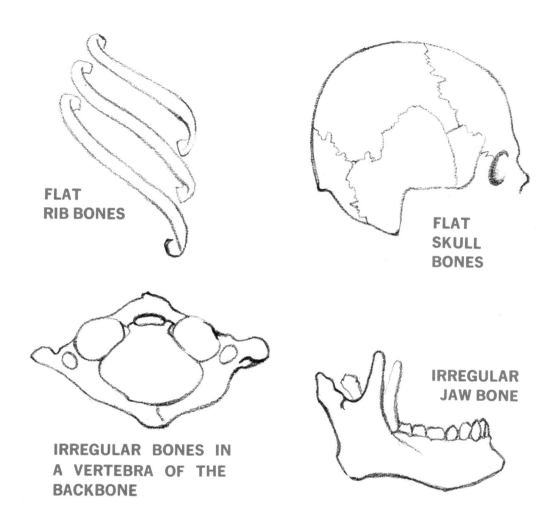

FLAT RIB BONES

FLAT SKULL BONES

IRREGULAR BONES IN A VERTEBRA OF THE BACKBONE

IRREGULAR JAW BONE

1. Long bones in the arms and legs

2. Short bones in the wrists and ankles

3. Flat bones in the ribs and several of the skullbones

4. Irregular bones in the backbone and jaw.

Any break in a bone is called a *fracture*. Fractures happen so often that practically everyone has had at least one.

Bone is brittle, and so it can break rather easily from a blow or fall. Because it is natural to stop a fall with outstretched hands, the commonest fracture is a "tipped-back" break of the wrist. This is called a *Colles fracture*, after Abraham Colles, an Irish surgeon who lived more than a hundred years ago.

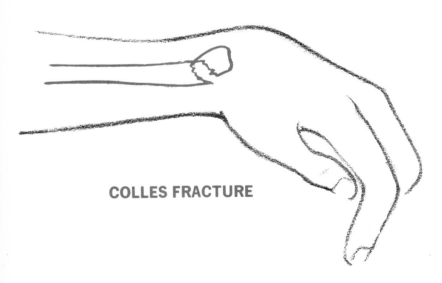

COLLES FRACTURE

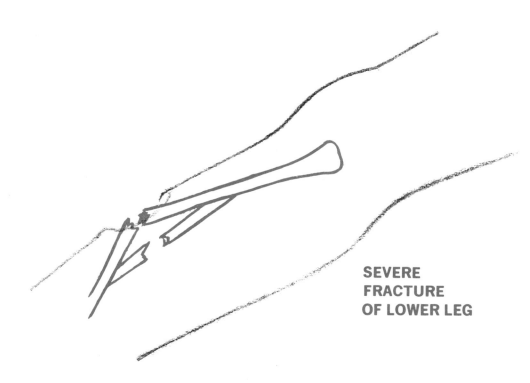

SEVERE
FRACTURE
OF LOWER LEG

Another extremely common fracture is a broken collarbone. It may break if you fall too hard on your hand or shoulder while playing basketball or skating. A shinbone break, or a leg break near the ankle, is also common. The signs of a broken bone are pain, swelling, and bruising. In a severe fracture the bone may come through the skin.

Although a bone can break, it can also do a remarkable job of mending and healing itself. Self-healing begins at the moment of fracture.

This is how a bone heals. First, the broken blood vessels at the place of fracture contract, which stops the flow of blood. Then *platelets*, an important part of the blood, gather around the break in the bone. (Platelets have their name because they are shaped like tiny plates. They live for only two to four days!)

Platelets help to repair leaks. They burst apart, and their chemicals make a protein that seals the leak. These platelets cause the blood around the break to thicken or clot. The clot stops the flow of blood from the wounded bone.

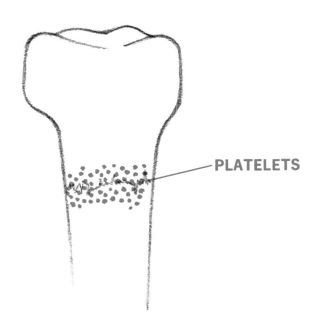

PLATELETS

EVANSTON PUBLIC LIBRARY
CHILDREN'S DEPARTMENT
1703 ORRINGTON AVENUE
EVANSTON, ILLINOIS 60201

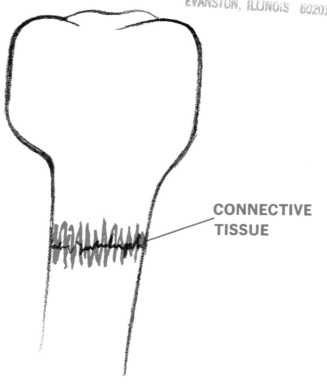

CONNECTIVE
TISSUE

In a few days minerals from the sharp ends of the broken bone are absorbed into the bloodstream. This leaves the ends soft and rubbery.

At the same time, pieces or fibers of *connective tissue* (the tissue that connects parts of the body) move to the place of the fracture. They grow through the clot and the fibers begin to hold the fractured pieces of bone together.

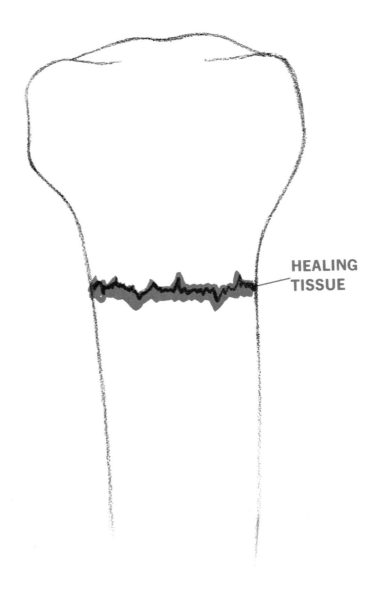

HEALING TISSUE

Inside this healing tissue is a special kind of cell. It is called an *osteoblast*, or "bone-maker." It deposits calcium and other minerals in the bone ends to strengthen them.

In two or three weeks soft, calcium-rich new bone, or *callus*, can be seen on X-rays. This closes the gap between the bone ends. When the callus hardens, the mended bone is ready again to take up its job of weight-bearing and support.

Often the healing is so well done that eventually an X-ray cannot detect an old fracture!

But this healing takes time. Bone may need months to heal. The deposit of enough calcium to strengthen and harden new bone is slow and gradual.

Bone cells grow and reproduce slowly because the blood supply to bone tissue is not as good as to other tissues.

OSTEOBLASTS

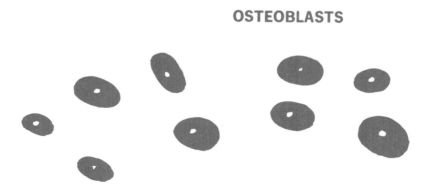

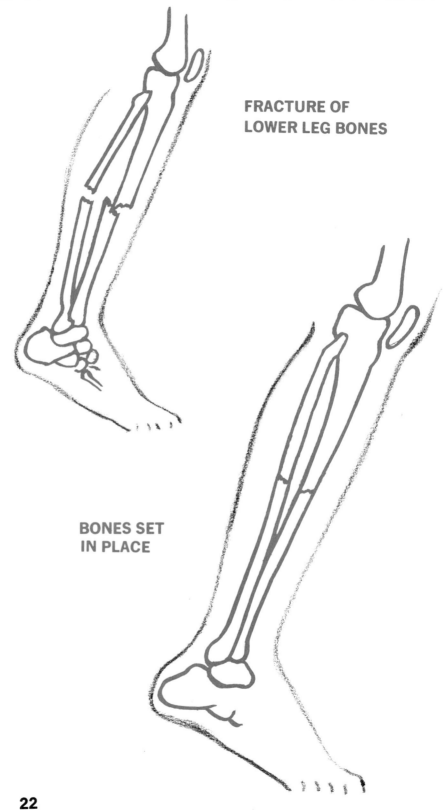

**FRACTURE OF
LOWER LEG BONES**

**BONES SET
IN PLACE**

In most cases, before a fracture begins to heal, the broken ends must be put back, or "set," in their proper position by a doctor. The ends are then held absolutely rigid by either plaster casts, metal plates, pins, or screws. The basic method of bone-setting has not changed for hundreds of years.

Young bones (like yours) are less brittle than the bones of an adult. Because your bones bend a little, your body can take a fall on the sidewalk or the ball field much more easily.

A long-bone fracture, where the bone bends rather than breaks completely, is called a "green-stick" fracture, because it looks like the splitting you see when you try to remove a branch from a growing bush.

GREEN-STICK FRACTURE

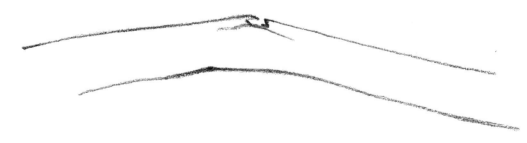

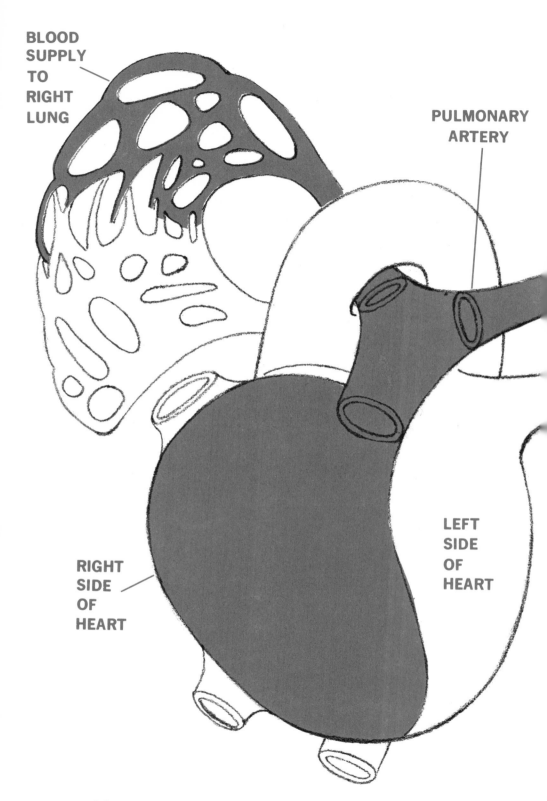

BLOOD
SUPPLY
TO
RIGHT
LUNG

PULMONARY
ARTERY

RIGHT
SIDE
OF
HEART

LEFT
SIDE
OF
HEART

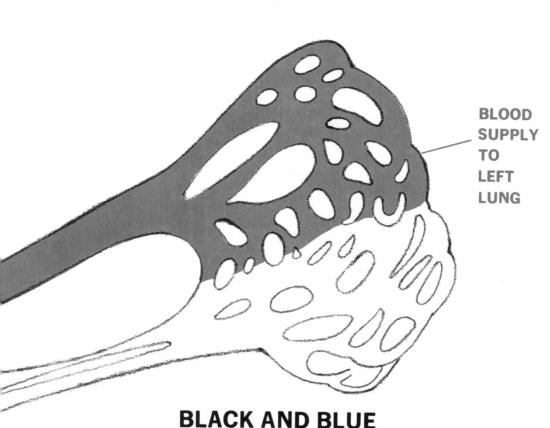

BLACK AND BLUE

Billions of blood cells are being pumped through you right this minute. Your heart pumps blood throughout the body. The blood travels through blood vessels called *arteries* and *veins*.

The arteries carry blood from the heart to the cells in every part of the body. In this way food dissolved in the blood is carried to the cells. Wastes from the cells are dissolved in the blood, and the veins carry this blood back from the cells to the heart.

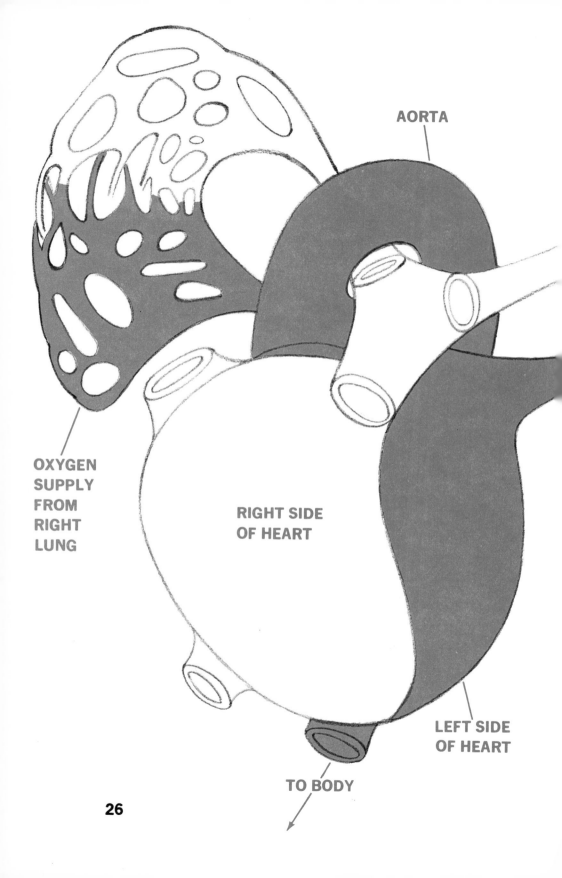

AORTA

OXYGEN
SUPPLY
FROM
RIGHT
LUNG

RIGHT SIDE
OF HEART

LEFT SIDE
OF HEART

TO BODY

26

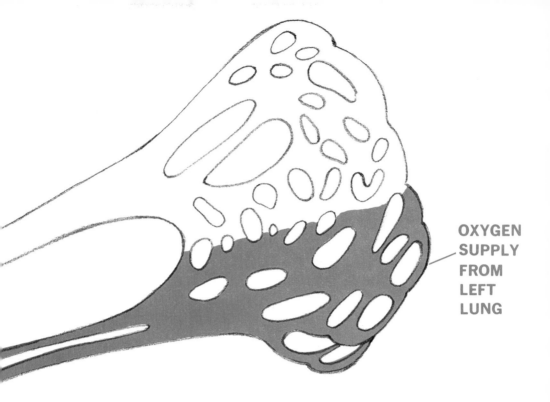

OXYGEN
SUPPLY
FROM
LEFT
LUNG

From the heart the blood goes to the lungs. There the waste gas, *carbon dioxide*, is removed and *oxygen* is added to the blood.

The blood then returns to the heart, where it is pumped out again to all of the body cells. Eight pints of blood keep going around and around.

The blood makes thousands of round trips every day. In a minute-long journey it supplies the needs of a fantastic number of different cells.

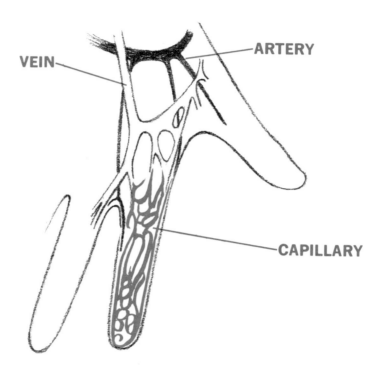

VEIN

ARTERY

CAPILLARY

The tiniest blood vessels in the body are called *capillaries*. They connect the arteries to the veins. Look at the palm of your hand and you can see the pinkish color of the tiny blood vessels showing through the skin.

When you get a "black-and-blue" bruise, these capillaries under the skin have been injured and broken. Blood leaks from the damaged capillaries and lies loose in the skin tissues. The color of the blood changes from red, to purple, to blue, to green, and finally to yellow.

A "black eye" is also a bruise. The blood capillaries around the eye break when the eye is struck. The tissues become baggy and swollen because an unusual amount of blood and fluid leak into them. This makes a bruise around the eye much more colorful than other injuries.

A "bump on the head," from either a blow or a fall, is a bruise, too. Blood and fluid leak from the damaged cells into the hurt area. Because of the tightness and closeness of the skin to the skullbone, the swelling is limited in its spreading. This is the "bump."

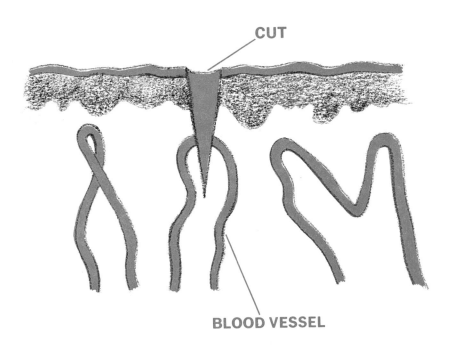

CUT

BLOOD VESSEL

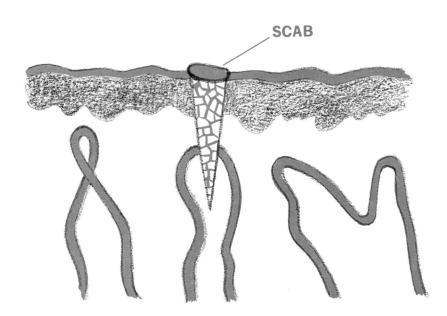

SCAB

30

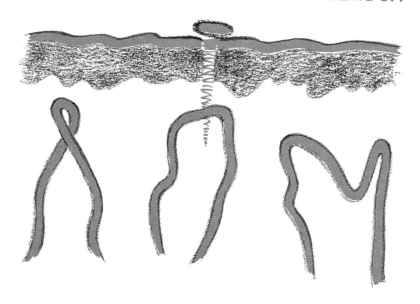

CUTS AND NOSEBLEEDS

Cuts usually bleed quite a bit. This is because the blood vessels have been cut across by a sharp-cutting object, such as a knife, a razor, or broken glass.

These wounds seldom become infected because very little skin tissue is destroyed and exposed. Also, the instant flow of blood from the cut washes out most of the foreign material.

31

Clotted blood forms on either side of the cut (see pages 18-19). This closes the cut, and blood cannot flow past it. The clot hardens and forms a crust on the skin. This crust is called a *scab*.

Later, as the cut heals, the area of clotted blood begins to shrink. The sides of the cut start to pull together. Cells of connective tissue move into the clot. Skin cells grow from either side of the cut to join at the center. When the tissue is healed, the scab falls off.

Sometimes the skin cells do not join perfectly, and this leaves a *scar*. But most times, the healing is complete. For example, when a fingertip is injured, even the fingertip *whorls* will grow back in their original pattern.

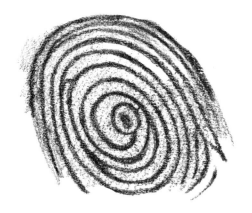

A *nosebleed* is also caused by damage to the small blood vessels. It is commonly caused by a blow or from nose-picking or other irritation. Five arteries meet in the nose passages, so there is an abundant supply of blood. It is no wonder that a nosebleed is a common occurrence.

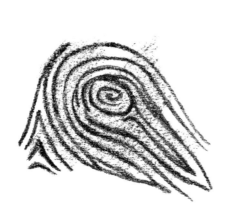

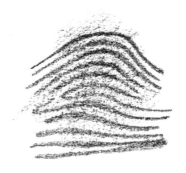

FINGERTIP WHORLS

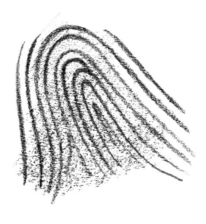

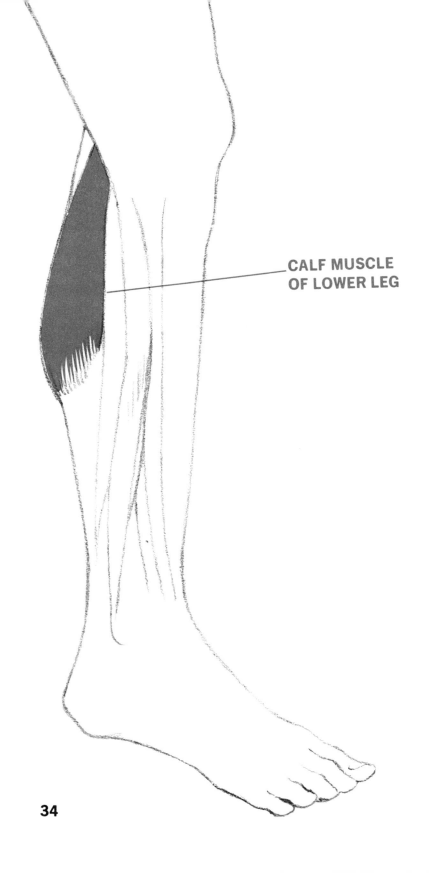

**CALF MUSCLE
OF LOWER LEG**

MUSCLES, SPRAINS, CRAMPS, SPASMS, AND NERVE INJURIES

When you have *muscle pain*, it is very likely brought on by strain or overuse of that muscle.

You often feel sore the day after overworking some part of your body, perhaps by playing too much tennis or shoveling too much snow.

Athletes sometimes overwork a leg or arm muscle. This puts too much strain and stress on the muscle and it tightens up. This is called a "charley horse," after the lame old nag who was overworked pulling the family wagon in the early days of this century. "Charley horse" was first used in baseball slang. It usually disappears after a few days—when the muscle, or muscles, are rested and relax again.

A *sprained ankle* is caused by twisting the foot while walking, running, or jumping on uneven ground. This pulls muscles and ligaments beyond their limits and brings immediate pain and swelling. If the ankle is strapped in place for about two weeks, the ligaments and muscles replace damaged cells and heal themselves.

A *cramp* is a sudden tightening of a muscle or muscles which causes sharp pain. It is also called a *spasm* of the muscle. A cramp comes from overusing the muscle or from chemical imbalances in the body.

A *stiff neck* is caused by a muscle spasm brought on by using the neck muscles too much or sitting in a draft. It can also occur when air-conditioning is too cold or drafty.

A "stitch in the side" is a muscle spasm, too.

The *dislocation* of a shoulder is a frequent injury in sports. The "head," or top, of the upper arm bone becomes separated from the shoulder bone. It is the only major joint in the body that is not really interlocked.

SPRAINED ANKLE

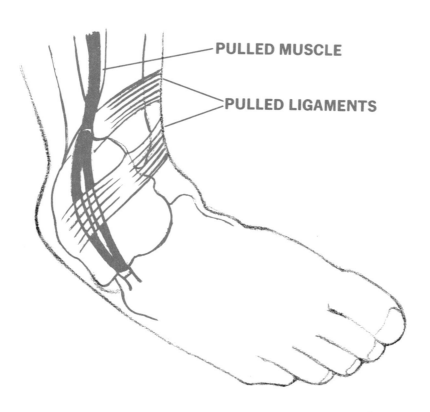

PULLED MUSCLE

PULLED LIGAMENTS

If the muscles that hold the shoulder joint in place have been injured, they go into spasm. They must be pulled and put back into place. The muscles have to be held that way until they relax again and recover from their injury. Because of this, the shoulder area is taped up to keep the bones in place. The bones in turn keep the muscles in place.

The *solar plexus* is the nerve center that controls your breathing. It is a network of nerves located at the pit of your stomach. When you are hit in the solar plexus, you lose the involuntary or unconscious control of breathing. Until the muscles and nerves recover from the shock of the blow, your "wind is knocked out."

Hitting your "funny bone" is quite painful. The *ulnar nerve* runs the whole length of your arm. Like most nerves, it is well protected by layers of muscle, except at that one point where it crosses the elbow just beneath the skin. So, when it is hit, the nerve carries its message of "Ouch!" along the spinal cord in the backbone to the brain. Your brain sends a message back to the elbow to move away fast. This exchange of signals happens in a fraction of a second, without you consciously deciding to move your elbow.

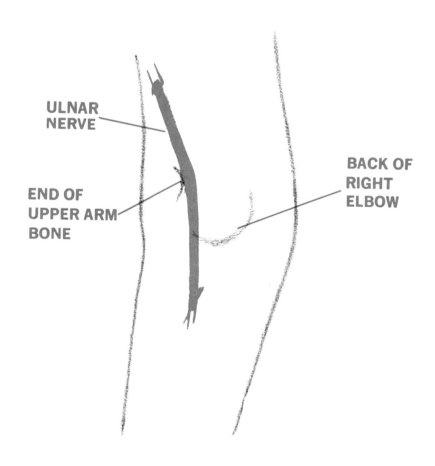

ULNAR NERVE

END OF UPPER ARM BONE

BACK OF RIGHT ELBOW

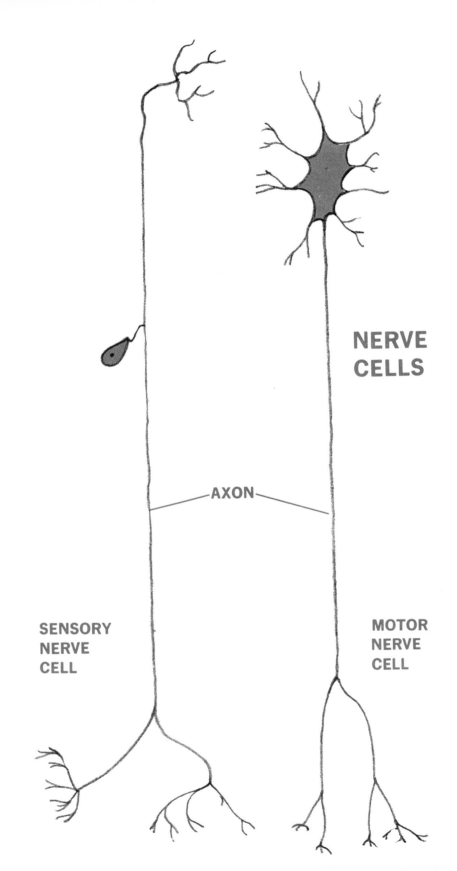

NERVE
CELLS

AXON

SENSORY
NERVE
CELL

MOTOR
NERVE
CELL

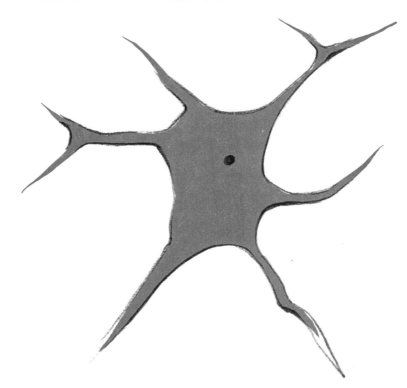

SPEAKING OF NERVES

What makes your elbow move away from something that hits it? What makes your stomach muscles and breathing muscles work? Why do your leg muscles turn right and left?

The answer is *nerve cells*. They control everything you do, every second of your life. When you decide to do something, nerve cells carry the message from your brain to the hundreds of muscles in your body (motor nerve cells), and they carry messages back (sensory nerve cells).

With your nerve cells you think, hear, taste, smell, feel pain, and do everyting in your life. They keep working even when you are asleep.

Nerve cells are a special shape that is different from other tissue cells. They have long, thin extensions called *axons* along which the messages from the brain travel.

These messages travel first to your *spinal cord*. This is a cable of very thin nerve cells, which is protected and enclosed by your backbone, or *spine*. More than four million nerve cells lie side by side. They whiz their messages back and forth, second after second, day and night. From the spinal cord the messages go to all parts of the body.

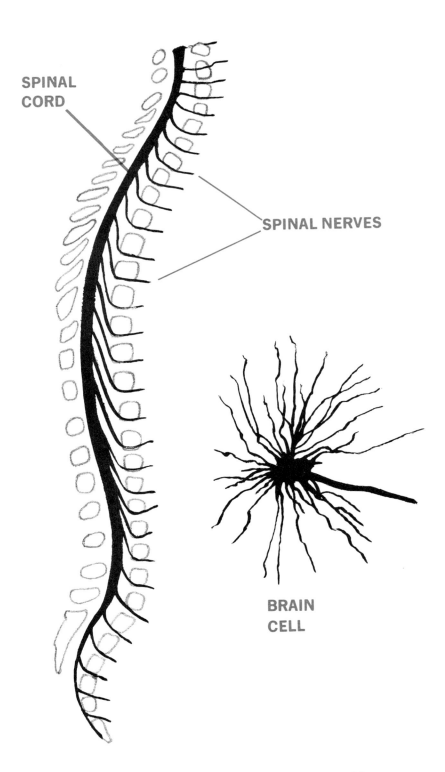

SPINAL
CORD

SPINAL NERVES

BRAIN
CELL

43

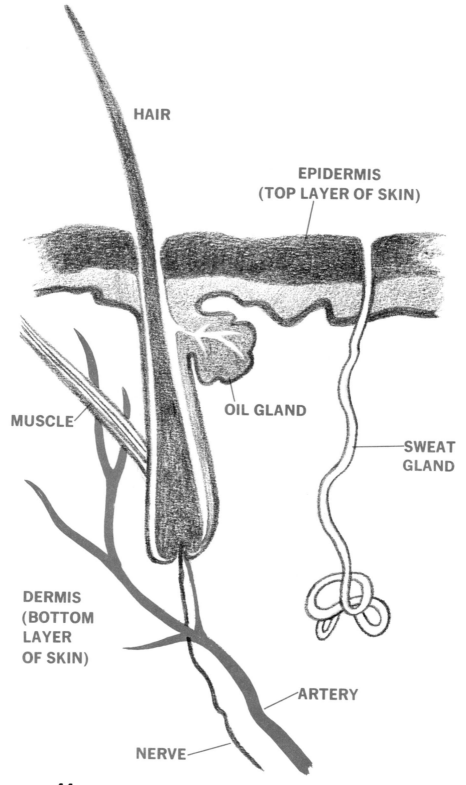

HAIR

EPIDERMIS
(TOP LAYER OF SKIN)

OIL GLAND

MUSCLE

SWEAT
GLAND

DERMIS
(BOTTOM
LAYER
OF SKIN)

ARTERY

NERVE

44

SKINNED KNEES, WARTS, AND SUNBURNS

Millions of cells make up the skin. It is a waterproof covering which prevents your body from drying out. (Your body is made up of 60 percent water.)

The skin has many nerve endings which receive and record all kinds of *stimuli*, such as heat or pressure, from outside the body.

The skin gives off heat when the body or its surroundings are hot, and keeps heat in the body when it is cold. In this way it helps regulate the body's temperature. The skin protects the body against external injury and disease-causing foreign bodies.

The skin can replace itself after injury or infection has destroyed its cells. At no point is it more than three-sixteenths of an inch thick, but it is composed of several layers of tissue.

The *epidermis*, or outer part of the skin, is made up of two to four layers, depending on the part of the body. The *dermis*, or inner part of the skin, has two layers. Cells produced in the bottom layer of the epidermis constantly push upward to replace the dead and dying cells above.

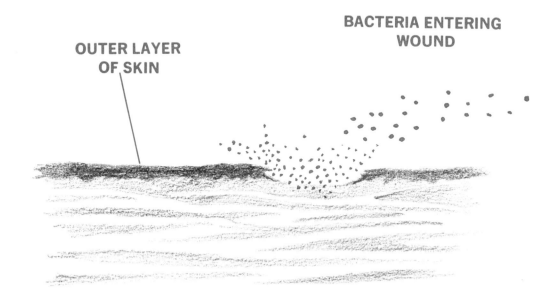

BACTERIA ENTERING WOUND

OUTER LAYER OF SKIN

The commonest of all skin disorders is *dandruff*. Loose flakes of skin form on the scalp and fall out when the hair is brushed or combed. They lie on the shoulders like a powder. These flakes are merely particles of the discarded upper layers of skin.

Hives are skin swellings that itch a lot. They may be caused by an allergy—an unusually sensitive reaction of the body to certain foods or drugs. They may also be caused by stings from nettles, jellyfish, or insects. Even emotional upsets can cause hives.

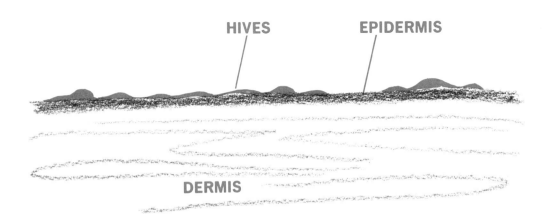

HIVES · EPIDERMIS · DERMIS

Fingernails and toenails are hard, tough skin cells made from a substance called *keratin*. They protect the tips of your fingers and toes. An "ingrown nail" digs into the flesh which surrounds it and damages the cells. This causes infection. An ingrown fingernail is caused by a naturally occurring, extra-curved nail. An ingrown toenail can be caused by the same thing, or by tight shoes or an overlapping toe.

"Losing a nail" means that serious injury has been done to the cells at the root of the nail. This root, or *matrix*, has to repair itself and grow a new nail.

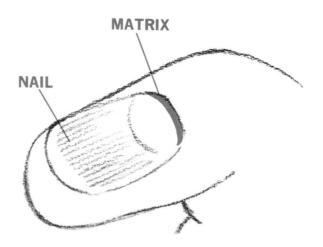

MATRIX

NAIL

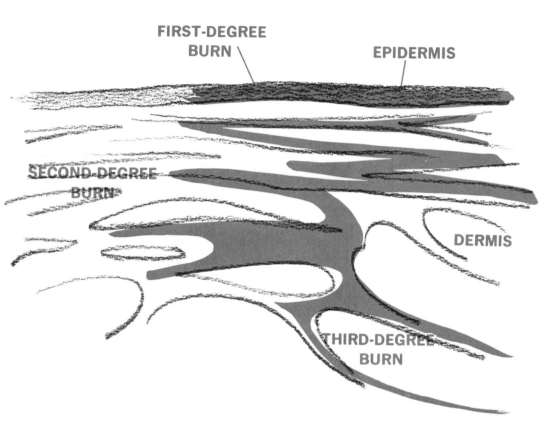

FIRST-DEGREE BURN

EPIDERMIS

SECOND-DEGREE BURN

DERMIS

THIRD-DEGREE BURN

BURNS

When you burn yourself, your skin cells are destroyed. A "first-degree" burn is mild damage to the top layers of skin. A "second-degree" burn is deeper damage to lower layers of the skin. A "third-degree" burn means destruction of the full thickness of the skin.

There is another kind of burn—a *sun-burn*. It is caused by overexposure to the sun. Your skin produces a certain amount of *melanin*, a dark pigment which absorbs the sun's ultraviolet rays. It is in the bottom layer of the epidermis.

Cells called *melanocytes* produce this pigment. More melanocytes are produced in the skin upon exposure to sunlight. Then the skin darkens, and you tan. But if you expose yourself too long to the sun's rays, not enough melanocytes can be produced to give protection, and you burn. Small groups of melanocytes produce islands of pigment called "freckles."

The excess ultraviolet rays of the sun

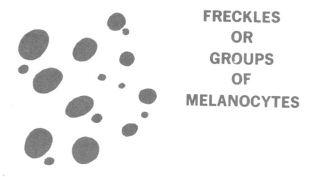

FRECKLES
OR
GROUPS
OF
MELANOCYTES

also cause the release of a chemical in the skin. This chemical makes the blood vessels swell, and the skin becomes red and sore.

Persons vary greatly in their reaction and sensitivity to ultraviolet rays. Blondes and redheads usually cannot take as much exposure as brunettes. This is because they do not have enough melanocytes in their skin.

Even on a cloudy day, enough ultraviolet rays can pass through the clouds to cause a burn. Reflections from snow, sand, water, or ice greatly increase the chance of getting burned.

If you expose yourself to the sun gradually, you can prevent sunburn. It is most important to avoid a long first exposure to the sun. If you are a brunette, start out with two 15- to 20-minute periods of strong sunlight the first day. Take two 30- to 45-minute periods on the second day, and increase the time gradually.

Blondes and redheads should begin their schedules with 5 to 10 minutes of exposure.

They should also use protective hats, clothing, or beach umbrellas.

A *blister* from a burn, or a badly fitting shoe, really guards the body. The epidermis swells up like a plastic cover to protect the underlying tissue from exposure to germs. Never break a blister. Let it do its job; it will collapse and wear off after your finger or toe is healed.

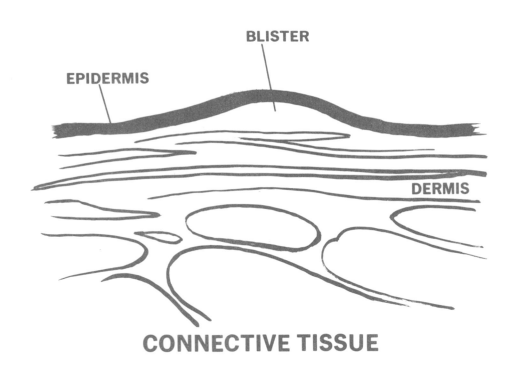

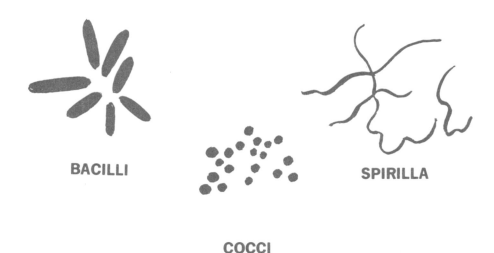

BACILLI

COCCI

SPIRILLA

INFECTIOUS DISEASES

Bacteria are made up of single cells. They are smaller than yeasts but larger than viruses. Some produce disease, some are harmless, some are useful (for instance, the bacteria in the soil of the earth help the growth of plants and trees).

Bacteria are classified according to their shape: *bacilli* are like rods; *cocci* are round; and *spirilla* are wavy.

Viruses are usually too small to be seen under an ordinary microscope. Viruses cause such diseases as influenza, measles, mumps, polio, smallpox, yellow fever, and chicken pox. Viruses also cause the common cold.

Bacteria and viruses, which are both also called "germs," invade the body from outside and cause infectious diseases. These diseases usually spread by "droplet infection." Tiny, tiny drops carrying germs are coughed or sneezed into the air by someone already suffering from the disease. These droplets can carry germs at least 10 to 15 feet!

The body deals with infection in many ways, but the main weapons are *antibodies* (special proteins in the blood serum) and the white blood cells. Antibodies work chemically against the germs. The white cells surround and destroy them after they have been attacked by the antibodies.

FIRST AID

The many, many millions of different cells in your body work, protect, heal, and provide food and energy to it year after year. Sometimes they need help to do these jobs—to help your body repair itself.

There are things that *you* can do. First aid is the way you can help a person who is hurt. It can be for any kind of minor wound or injury: cuts, bruises, burns, or broken bones.

Very often it is the only kind of help needed. However, if the wound is serious, a doctor should take over where the first aid leaves off.

Acne: The entire body, especially the face, must be kept clean by frequent washing.

Steamed towels are helpful in softening some dirt plugs in the skin glands. Any further treatment, such as the application of medicine or the control of diet, should be under the supervision of a doctor.

Black-and-blue bruises: Put ice cubes or a cold washcloth directly on the bruise. This reduces swelling and relieves pain. It also helps to prevent discoloration of the skin in a "black eye."

Blackheads and pimples: Keep the skin absolutely clean by frequent washing. Steamed cloths help bring the dirt of the blackhead to the surface of the skin and help bring a pimple "to a head," to get rid of the infection.

Boils: Boils should be protected from irritation, and moist heat should be applied from time to time. The skin must be kept very clean by frequent washing with soap and water. Your doctor may give you special ointments. But it is very important that you keep your skin clean.

Bump on the head: Apply ice cubes or a cold cloth. The swelling will go down in a short time.

Burns: For a simple burn without blisters, run cold water over the burned place at once. You can also put ice cubes on it. Continue until the pain goes away.

If the burn is blistered or deep, or covers a rather large area of the body, a doctor should examine it right away.

Cramp: Massage the painful muscle, and stretch it. For example, to relax a cramped calf muscle, straighten your knee and press your toes upwards.

Cuts: First, stop the bleeding by putting pressure on the cut with a cold wet tissue or compress. Then wash the cut with soap and water, under a running faucet, if possible. Put on a Bandaid and press down on the cut again. If it is a large or deep cut, go to a doctor right away.

Dislocated shoulder: The injured part should be made as comfortable as possible. Call a doctor.

Hives: There are so many possible causes of hives that you should simply see your doctor right away.

Loss of a nail: Put on a loose bandage or Bandaid to protect the tender under-skin from dirt or injury. Elevate the hand to ease the pain.

Nosebleed: Stand with your head bent forward, and pinch the soft end of the nose with your thumb and first finger. If you have a severe nosebleed and tip your head backwards, the blood could trickle into your throat and cause you to choke.

Skinned knee: The skinning needs a thorough cleansing with soap and water to remove the bacteria or dirt. Then apply a first-aid cream and put on a sterile, or antiseptic, clean bandage to protect the injury.

Sprained ankle: Immediately put on ice cubes, and stay off feet for 24 hours. Keep foot elevated. After 12 hours apply low heat; then put on an elastic or Ace bandage.

Sunburn: There are many creams, lotions, and oils to help prevent sunburn. They will help give you a healthful "tan." If you do get sunburned, calamine lotion is soothing. If it is a very bad sunburn, and is serious, see a doctor right away.

INDEX

(Figures in italics indicate pages upon which illustrations occur.)